LUBY FRENCH DOOR TOASTER OVEN COOKBOOK

EASY, DELICIOUS, AFFORDABLE AND SIMPLE RECIPES TO BAKE, TOAST, BROIL WHICH ANYONE CAN COOK.

DANA REED

CONTENTS

CHICKEN AND POULTRY

SNACKS AND APPETIZERS

VEGAN AND VEGETARIAN

BEANS AND EGGS

DESSERTS AND SNACKS

INTRODUCTION

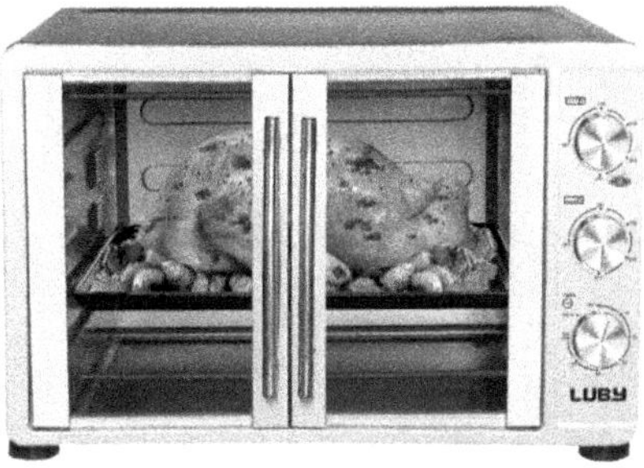

The Luby French Door Toaster Oven is possibly one of the most versatile and advanced Toaster Oven out there in the market. Long gone are the days where you had to purchase multiple appliances for baking, toasting, or broiling! With the Luby French Door Toaster Oven, you will be able to do all of them using just a single appliance!

This will not only save up lots of space in your kitchen but will also save you from burning a pocket in your hole. And let's not forget the fantastic French Door Style design of the product, which takes very minimal space even when you open the door.

With this particular appliance, you will be able to effortlessly

Bake, Toast, or Broil your meals to absolute perfection and with ease!

The Oven has a usable interior dimension of 16-3/8W x 15-7/8D x 8-1/2H

This gives you more than enough capacity to bake a 14-inch pizza, roast an almost 20 pounds turkey, bake a cake for the whole family, or even bake 24 cups of muffin all in one go!

The ability to place your racks in both an upper and lower position and set temperature for the both of the racks individually further increases the internal space's usability!

This particular handbook is designed to give you an overview of the appliance and cover the basic fundamentals required to use this appliance properly.

In this book, you will find:

•A brief explanation of the core features of the appliance

•Step by step guide on how to keep your appliance clean and maintain it for prolonged usability

•The advantages of owning a Luby French Door Toaster Oven

•The primary features and functions of the Luby French Door Toaster Oven

And lot more!

And once you are done with the basics and have a good understanding, you will have the opportunity to explore a plethora of absolutely hand-picked and fool-proof collection of 60+ mouthwatering and inspiring recipes that will encourage you to use the appliance even more and discover your very own culinary masterpiece.

All of the recipes and carefully divided into individual categories so that you can find what you are looking for with absolute ease.

So, what are you waiting for? Grab your copy right now and start exploring a new culinary world with the amazing Luby French Door Toaster Oven and impress all of your friends and family with dazzling and heartwarming meals!

What Is It?

The Luby French Door Toaster Oven is possibly one of the most stylish looking convection ovens out there designed to perform multiple under the singlehood. With this appliance, you can seamlessly Bake, Broil and Toast your meals to perfection and with absolute ease.

The appliance is built from the ground up using extremely high-quality stainless steel, giving this Oven a very sleek and modern look. Both of the doors of the Oven open very easily by just pulling a single door by one hand.

The appliances work on a very meticulously crafted convection baking technology that allows your meals to cook faster while producing a very fine and brown texture.

The Oven's Extra-large interior allows you to bake a 14 inch sized pizza or even a 20-pound turkey with absolute ease!

If you are looking for the perfect Oven that can move Bake, Broil, and Toast effortlessly, then this is the one that you need!

BRUNCHES

1

APPLE OAT CUPS

Prep Time: 10 minutes/ **Cook Time** 30 minutes/ **Serves:** 12

Ingredients :

•3 cups oats, old-fashioned

•2 eggs

•½ cup apple sauce

•2 teaspoons baking powder

•2 tablespoons brown sugar

•1 cup milk 1 and ¼ cups apples, peel and diced

•2 teaspoons vanilla

•2 teaspoons cinnamon, grounded

•¼ teaspoon salt

Directions :

1.Preheat your Oven t0 350 degrees F

2.Spray 12-cups muffin tin with cooking spray

3.Keep it aside

4.Add oats, cinnamon, brown sugar, baking powder, and salt into a bowl

5.Mix them well and set aside

6.Add vanilla, applesauce, milk, and whisked egg in a large bowl

7.Add oat mixture into the egg mixture
8.Stir well
9.Stuff the mixture into the muffin tray
10.Place it into your over the rack
11.Bake for 30 minutes
12.Serve and enjoy!

Nutritional Contents:

•Calories: 122
•Carbohydrate: 21.5 g
•Protein: 4.3 g
•Fat: 2.5 g

2

HEALTHY OAT MUFFINS

Prep Time: 10 minutes/ **Cook Time** 20 minutes/ **Serves:** 12

Ingredients :

•1 cup oats

•½ cup plain yogurt

•2 teaspoons baking powder

•1 cup butternut squash puree

•1 cup flour

•½ cup maple syrup

•1/3 cup olive oil

•1 tablespoon pumpkin pie spice

•2 eggs

•1 teaspoon vanilla

•½ teaspoon of sea salt

Directions :

1.Preheat your Oven t0 390 degrees F

2.Spray 12-cups muffin tray with cooking spray

3.Keep it aside

4.Take a large bowl and add yogurt, butternut squash puree; whisk the egg with vanilla, oil, and maple syrup

5.Take another bowl and add pumpkin pie spice, oats, flour, and salt

6.Mix them well

7.Add flour mixture into your egg mixture

8.Stir well to combine

9.Pour the batter into the prepared muffin tray

10.Place the pan onto the oven rack

11.Bake for 20 minutes

12.Serve and enjoy!

Nutritional Contents:

•Calories: 167

•Carbohydrate: 22.9 g

•Protein: 3.5 g

•Fat: 7.1 g

3

BAKED CINNAMON OATMEAL

Prep Time: 10 minutes/ **Cook Time** 30 minutes/ **Serves:** 8

Ingredients :

•3 cups oats, rolled

•½ maple syrup

•1 and ½ cups of almond milk

•1 teaspoon cinnamon, grounded

•2 eggs

•1 teaspoon vanilla

•1 and ½ teaspoons baking powder

•¼ cup butter, melted

•Pinch of salt

Directions :

1.Preheat your Oven t0 350 degrees F

2.Take a bowl and add vanilla, baking powder, butter, maple syrup, whisked egg with almond milk and salt into it

3.Add oats and mix them well

4.Greased your baking pan

5.Pour the mixture into that baking pan

6.Place the baking pan onto the oven rack

7.Bake for 30 minutes

8.Serve and enjoy!

Nutritional Contents:

•Calories: 341

•Carbohydrate: 37.3 g

•Protein: 6.5 g

•Fat: 19.6 g

4

EASY LEMON COOKIES

Prep Time: 10 minutes/ **Cook Time** 11 minutes/ **Serves:** 12

Ingredients :

•1 egg yolk

•½ teaspoon baking powder

•¼ teaspoon baking soda

•1 lemon zest

•2 teaspoons vanilla

•1 tablespoon brown sugar

•1 cup of sugar

•1 and ¼ cups flour

•½ cup butter softened

•¼ teaspoon salt

Directions :

1.Preheat your Oven t0 350 degrees F

2.Take a bowl and add flour, baking powder, baking soda, and salt to it

3.Take another bowl and add butter, ¾ cup sugar, and brown sugar until you get a fluffy mixture

4.Add eggs, vanilla, and lemon zest

5.Beat until it combines well

6.Make 1 and ½ inch ball from the mixture

7.Roll into the remaining sugar and place onto the parchment-lined baking pan

8.Bake for 11 minutes

9.Once cooked, removed the pan and allow it to cool

10.Serve and enjoy!

Nutritional Contents:

•Calories: 187

•Carbohydrate: 27.6 g

•Protein: 1.7 g

•Fat: 8.2 g

5

CHOCOLATE CHIP COOKIES

Prep Time: 10 minutes/ **Cook Time** 8 minutes/ **Serves:** 30

Ingredients :

•12 ounces of chocolate chips

•2 cups self-rising flour

•1 egg

•1 teaspoon vanilla

•1 cup butter, softened

•½ cup brown sugar

•2/3 cup sugar

Directions :

1.Preheat your Oven t0 375 degrees F

2.Take a bowl and add egg, vanilla, and butter

3.Add brown sugar and sugar, beat until you get a creamy mixture

4.Add flour slowly and mix to combine

5.Add chocolate chips and stir well

6.Spoon out cookie dough onto the parchment-lined baking pan

7.Bake for 8-11 minutes

8.Once cooked, removed the pan and allow it to cool

9.Serve and enjoy!

Nutritional Contents:

•Calories: 174

•Carbohydrate: 19.9 g

•Protein: 0 g

•Fat: 9.7 g

6

CRUNCHY FLAX AND ALMOND CRACKERS

Prep Time: 15 minutes/ **Cook Time** 1 hour/ **Serves:** 20-24

Ingredients :

•½ cup almond flour

•1 tablespoon coconut flour

•½ cup ground flax seeds

•1 egg white

•2 tablespoons shelled hemp seeds

•2 tablespoons unsalted almond butter, melted

•¼ teaspoon sunflower seeds

Directions :

1.Preheat your Oven t0 300 degrees F in Bake mode

2.Line a baking sheet with parchment paper

3.Keep it aside

4.Take a bowl and add coconut flour, hemp seed, almond, flax seeds into the bowl

5.Mix them well

6.Add melted almond butter and egg, mix until combined

7.Transfer dough to a sheet of parchment paper and cover with another sheet of paper

8.Roll out dough and cut into crackers

9.Bake for 1 hour
10.Let them cool
11.Serve and enjoy!

Nutritional Contents:

•Calories: 00
•Carbohydrate: 1.2 g
•Protein: 2 g
•Fat: 6 g

7

MUSHROOM PIZZA

Prep Time: 10 minutes/ **Cook Time** 15 minutes/ **Serves:** 4

Ingredients :

•¾ pound Portobello mushrooms, stems removed

•½ cup cashew cheese

•2 cloves garlic, minced

•½ cup tomato puree

•2 tablespoons olive oil

•Salt and pepper, to taste

Directions :

1.Preheat your Oven t0 350 degrees F

2.Brush oil on the inverted side of the mushrooms

3.Then brush with sprinkle garlic and tomato puree

4.Add cashew cheese on top

5.Place it on a baking pan

6.Bake for 15 minutes

7.Serve and enjoy!

Nutritional Contents:

•Calories: 112

•Carbohydrate: 7 g

- Protein: 7 g
- Fat: 7 g

8

BAKED OATMEAL

Prep Time: 10 minutes/ **Cook Time** 20 minutes/ **Serves:** 6

Ingredients :

•2 cups oats, old fashioned

•1 cup strawberries, sliced

•1 egg

•1 and ½ teaspoon baking powder

•¼ cup maple syrup

•1 and ½ cups of almond milk

•½ teaspoon salt

Directions :

1.Preheat your Oven t0 375 degrees F

2.Add oats, baking powder, and salt into a bowl

3.Add egg, vanilla, maple syrup, and almond milk

4.Stir them well

5.Add strawberries and blueberries, stir it

6.Pour mixture into the baking dish

7.Place the pan onto the oven rack

8.Bake for 20 minutes

9.Serve and enjoy!

Nutritional Contents:

•Calories: 413

•Carbohydrate: 53.9 g

•Protein: 9.3 g

•Fat: 18.7 g

BEEF, PORK AND LAMB

9

AWESOME MEATBALLS

Prep Time: 10 minutes/ **Cook Time** 20 minutes/ **Serves:** 4

Ingredients :

•1 pound lamb, grounded

•1/4 teaspoon basil, dried

•1/4 teaspoon oregano, dried

•1 garlic clove, minced

•1/4 cup fresh cilantro, chopped

•1/4 cup raisins

•1/4 cup yogurt

•2 bread slices, cut into small pieces

•Salt and pepper

Directions :

1.Preheat your Oven t0 375 degrees F

2.Add all ingredients into the mixing bowl

3.Mix them well

4.Make balls from the meat mixture

5.Make sure the balls are in the same size

6.Place into the parchment-lined baking pan

7.Then bake for 20 minutes

8.Serve and enjoy!

Nutritional Contents:

•Calories: 263

•Carbohydrate: 10.9 g

•Protein: 33.4 g

•Fat: 8.7 g

10

SPINACH AND BEEF MEATBALLS

Prep Time: 10 minutes/ **Cook Time** 20 minutes/ **Serves:** 4

Ingredients :

•1 pound lean ground beef
•10 ounces spinach
•4 garlic cloves
•1 whole egg
•1/4 teaspoon oregano
•1/2 cup onion
•Pepper as needed

Directions :

1.Preheat your Toaster Oven to 375 degrees F in Bake mode
2.Take a bowl and add all the ingredients to it
3.Mix them by using your hands and roll into meatballs
4.Transfer them into a sheet tray
5.Bake for 20 minutes
6.Serve and enjoy!

Nutritional Contents:

•Calories: 37
•Carbohydrate: 2 g

- Protein: 1 g
- Fat: 3 g

11

RAVAGING BEEF POT ROAST

Prep Time: 10 minutes/ **Cook Time** 1 hour 15 minutes/ **Serves:** 4

Ingredients :

- 12 ounces beef stock
- 4 ounces mushrooms, sliced
- 3 and ½ pounds beef roast
- ½ cup Italian dressing, low sodium, and low fat
- 1-ounce onion soup mix

Directions :

1. Preheat your Toaster Oven to 300 degrees F in Bake Mode
2. Add onion soup mix, Italian dressing, and the stock into a bowl
3. Stir it slowly
4. Take a pan and put the beef roast
5. Add mushrooms, stock mix to the pan, and cover with foil
6. Bake for 1 hour and 15 minutes
7. Let the roast cool, then slice it
8. Serve and enjoy!

Nutritional Contents:

- Calories: 37
- Carbohydrate: 2 g
- Protein: 1 g
- Fat: 3 g

12

ALMOND PORK CHOPS

Prep Time: 10 minutes/ **Cook Time** 25 minutes/ **Serves:** 4

Ingredients:

- 1 tablespoon almond butter, divided
- 2 boneless pork chops
- pepper to taste
- 1 tablespoon dried Italian seasoning, low fat, and low sodium
- 1 tablespoon olive oil

Directions:

1.Preheat your Toaster Oven to 350 degrees F in Bake Mode

2.Pat pork chops dry with a paper towel and place them in a baking dish

3.Season with pepper and Italian seasoning

4.Drizzle olive oil over pork chops

5.Top each chop with ½ tablespoon almond butter

6.Bake for 25 minutes

7.Transfer pork chops on two plates and top with almond butter juice

8.Serve and enjoy!

Nutritional Contents:

- Calories: 37
- Fat: 3g
- Carbohydrates: 2g
- Protein: 1g

13

GROUND BEEF CASSEROLE

Prep Time: 10 minutes/ **Cook Time** 35 minutes/ **Serves:** 4

Ingredients:

•2 teaspoons onion flakes

•1 tablespoon gluten-free Worcestershire sauce

•2 pounds ground beef

•2 garlic clove, peeled and minced

•Salt and pepper to taste

•1 cup mozzarella cheese, shredded

•2 cups cheddar cheese, shredded

•1 cup Russian dressing

•2 tablespoons sesame seeds, toasted

•20 dill pickle slices

•1 romaine lettuce head, torn

Directions:

1.Take a pan and place it over medium heat

2.Add beef, onion flakes, Worcestershire sauce, salt, pepper, and garlic

3.Stir for 5 minutes

4.Transfer to a baking dish and add 1 cup of cheddar, mozzarella cheese, half of dressing

5.Stir and spread evenly. Arrange pickle slices on top

6.Sprinkle remaining cheddar and sesame seeds

7.Transfer to Toaster Oven and bake for 20 minutes at 350 degrees F in Bake Mode. Turn Toaster Oven to broil and broil for 5 minutes

8.Divide lettuce between serving platters and top with remaining dressing. Enjoy!

Nutritional Contents:

•Calories: 554

•Fat: 51g

•Carbohydrates: 5g

•Protein: 45g

FISH AND SEAFOOD

14

EASY GARLIC ALMOND BUTTER SHRIMP

Prep Time: 15 minutes/ **Cook Time** 30 minutes/ **Serves:** 4

Ingredients :

•4 pounds shrimp

•½ cup almond butter

•1 tablespoon lemon pepper seasoning

•1-2 tablespoons garlic, minced

•½ teaspoon garlic powder

Directions :

1.Preheat your toaster oven to 300 degrees F in Toast mode

2.Add garlic and almond butter into a bowl

3.Mix them well

4.Place shrimp in a pan and dot with almond butter garlic mix

5.Sprinkle lemon pepper and garlic powder

6.Bake for 30 minutes

7.Serve and enjoy!

Nutritional Contents:

•Calories: 749

•Carbohydrate: 7 g

•Protein: 74 g

•Fat: 30 g

15

SPICY BAKED COD

Prep Time: 15 minutes/ **Cook Time** 15 minutes/ **Serves:** 5

Ingredients :

•5 cod fillets

•2 tablespoons curry powder

•2 tablespoons olive oil

•2 tablcspoons plain yogurt, non-fat

•1 teaspoon ginger, grated

•1 teaspoon soy sauce

•2 and ½ teaspoon cayenne pepper

•1 teaspoon of rice wine vinegar

Directions :

1.Preheat your toaster oven to 400 degrees F in Bake mode

2.Add all ingredients except oil in a shallow dish

3.Mix them well and allow it to marinate for 1 hour

4.Grease cookie sheet with oil

5.Place cod filet on a prepared cookie sheet

6.Bake for 15 minutes

7.Serve and enjoy!

Nutritional Contents:

- Calories: 254
- Carbohydrate: 2 g
- Protein: 42 g
- Fat: 1 g

16

HEART-WARMING MEDI TILAPIA

Prep Time: 15 minutes/ **Cook Time** 15 minutes/ **Serves:** 4

Ingredients :

•2 tilapia fillets

•2 tablespoons kalamata olives, chopped and pitted

•3 tablespoons sun-dried tomatoes, packed in oil, drained and choppcd

•1 tablespoon capers, drained

•1 tablespoon oil from sun-dried tomatoes

Directions :

1.Preheat your toaster oven to 370 degrees F in Toast mode

2.Add tomatoes, capers, and olives into a small-sized bowl

3.Keep the mixture on the side

4.Take a baking sheet

5.Transfer the tilapia fillets and arrange them side by side

6.Drizzle olive oil all over them

7.Toast for 10-15 minutes

8.After 10 minutes, check the fish for a "Flaky" texture

9.Top the fish with tomato mixture

10.Serve and enjoy!

Nutritional Contents:

- Calories: 183
- Carbohydrate: 18 g
- Protein: 0 g
- Fat: 8 g

17

SPICY ROASTED SHRIMP

Prep Time: 10 minutes/ **Cook Time** 8 minutes/ **Serves:** 4

Ingredients :

•½ ounces large shrimp, peeled and deveined

•1 teaspoon low sodium coconut aminos

•½ tablespoon honey

•1 teaspoon parsley

•1 tablespoon lemon juice

•½ teaspoon olive oil

•Cooking spray as needed

Directions :

1.Preheat your toaster oven to 450 degrees F in Toast mode

2.Take a baking dish and grease it well

3.Mix in all the ingredients

4.Toss it

5.Transfer to Toaster Oven

6.Bake for 8 minutes until shrimp turn pink

7.Serve and enjoy!

Nutritional Contents:

•Calories: 284

•Carbohydrate: 1 g
•Protein: 32 g
•Fat: 18 g

18

LOVELY CALAMARI

Prep Time: 10 minutes + 1 hour marinating / **Cook Time** 10 minutes/ **Serves:** 4

Ingredients

•2 tablespoons extra virgin olive oil

•1 teaspoon chili powder

•½ teaspoon ground cumin

•Zest of 1 lime

•Juice of 1 lime

•Dash of sea sunflower seeds

•1 and ½ pounds squid, cleaned and split open, with tentacles cut into ½ inch rounds

•2 tablespoons cilantro, chopped

•2 tablespoons red bell pepper, minced

Directions:

1.Take a medium bowl and stir in olive oil, chili powder, cumin, lime zest, sea sunflower seeds, lime juice, and pepper

2.Add squid and let it marinade and stir to coat, coat and let it refrigerate for 1 hour

3.Preheat your Toaster Oven to broil

4.Arrange squid on a baking sheet, broil for 8 minutes turn once until tender

5.Garnish the broiled calamari with cilantro and red bell pepper

6.Serve and enjoy!

Nutritional Contents:

•Calories: 159

•Fat: 13g

•Carbohydrates: 12g

•Protein: 3g

19

PREMIUM ALMOND BUTTER SHRIMP

Prep Time: 10 minutes/ **Cook Time** 30 minutes/ **Serves:** 4

Ingredients

•4 pounds shrimp

•1-2 tablespoons garlic, minced

•½ cup almond butter

•1 tablespoon lemon pepper seasoning

•½ teaspoon garlic powder

Directions:

1.Preheat your toaster oven to 300 degrees F in Toast mode

2.Take a bowl and mix in garlic and almond butter

3.Place shrimp in a pan and dot with almond butter garlic mix

4.Sprinkle garlic powder and lemon pepper

5.Bake for 30 minutes

6.Enjoy!

Nutritional Contents:

•Calories: 749

•Fat: 30g

•Net Carbohydrates: 7g

•Protein: 74g

20

TILAPIA AND BROCCOLI MEAL

Prep Time: 10 minutes/ **Cook Time** 14 minutes/ **Serves:** 4

Ingredients

•6 ounce of tilapia, frozen

•1 tablespoon of almond butter

•1 tablespoon of garlic, minced

•1 teaspoon of lemon pepper seasoning

•1 cup of broccoli florets, fresh

Directions:

1.Preheat your toaster oven to 350 degrees Fahrenheit in bake mode

2.Add fish in aluminum foil packets.

3.Arrange broccoli around fish.

4.Sprinkle lemon pepper on top.

5.Close the packets and seal.

6.Bake for 14 minutes.

7.Take a bowl and add garlic and almond butter, mix well, and keep the mixture on the side.

8.Remove the packet from the Oven and transfer it to a platter.

9.Place almond butter on top of the fish and broccoli, serve and enjoy!

Nutritional Contents:

•Calories: 362

•Fat: 25g

•Net Carbohydrates: 2g

•Protein: 29g

21

LOVELY DIJON FISH

Prep Time: 10 minutes/ **Cook Time** 12 minutes/ **Serves:** 4

Ingredients:

- 1 perch, flounder, or sole fish florets
- 1 tablespoon Dijon mustard
- 1 and ½ teaspoon lemon juice
- 1 teaspoon low sodium Worcestershire sauce, low sodium
- 2 tablespoons Italian seasoned bread crumbs
- 1 almond butter-flavored cooking spray

Directions

1.Preheat your Toaster Oven to 450 degrees Fahrenheit in Bake Mode

2.Take an 11 x 7-inch baking dish and arrange your fillets carefully

3.Take a small-sized bowl and add lemon juice, Worcestershire sauce, mustard and mix it well

4.Pour the mix over your fillet

5.Sprinkle a good amount of breadcrumbs

6.Bake for 12 minutes until fish flakes off easily

7.Cut the fillet in half portions and enjoy!

Nutritional Contents:

•Calories: 284

•Fat: 18g

•Carbohydrates: 1g

•Protein: 32g

CHICKEN AND POULTRY

22

JUICY CHICKEN DRUMSTICKS

Prep Time: 10 minutes/ **Cook Time** 45 minutes/ **Serves:** 6

Ingredients :

•6 chicken legs

•2 tablespoons olive oil

•1 and ½ teaspoons onion powder

•1 teaspoon garlic powder

•¼ cup of soy sauce

•½ teaspoon paprika

•½ teaspoon oregano

•½ teaspoon salt

•½ teaspoon pepper

Directions :

1.Preheat your Oven t0 375 degrees F

2.Add chicken legs and the rest of the ingredients into the zip-lock bag

3.Seal the bag and shake well

4.Place it into the refrigerator for 1 hour

5.Place rack onto a baking tray

6.Arrange marinated chicken legs onto the rack

7.Place it into your Oven

8.Bake for 45 minutes
9.Serve and enjoy!

Nutritional Contents:

•Calories: 315
•Carbohydrate: 1.9 g
•Protein: 30.5 g
•Fat: 20.1 g

23

CRISPY CHICKEN WINGS

Prep Time: 10 minutes/ **Cook Time** 50 minutes/ **Serves:** 6

Ingredients :

•2 pounds of chicken wings

•1 teaspoon Italian seasoning

•1 tablespoon baking powder

•1 teaspoon garlic powder

•1 teaspoon paprika, smoked

•1 teaspoon salt

•1/4 teaspoon pepper

Directions :

1.Preheat your Oven t0 425 degrees F

2.Take a mixing bowl and add chicken wings and the rest of the ingredients into it

3.Toss it well

4.Place rack onto a baking tray

5.Arrange chicken wings onto the rack

6.Insert into the Oven

7.Bake for 30 minutes

8.Flip your chicken wings and bake for 20 minutes more

9.Serve and enjoy!

Nutritional Contents:
•Calories: 295
•Carbohydrate: 1.9 g
•Protein: 43.9 g
•Fat: 11.5 g

24

LEMON PEPPER CHICKEN WINGS

Prep Time: 10 minutes/ **Cook Time** 25 minutes/ **Serves:** 6

Ingredients :

•1 and ½ pounds chicken wings

•6 tablespoons butter, melted

•3 tablespoons olive oil

•½ lemon juice

•2 tablespoons honey

•½ teaspoon pepper

•Salt

Directions :

1.Preheat your Oven t0 425 degrees F

2.Brush the chicken wings with oil

3.Season with salt and pepper

4.Place rack onto a baking tray

5.Arrange chicken wings onto the rack

6.Insert into the Oven

7.Bake for 25 minutcs

8.Brush chicken wings with honey mixture

9.Serve and enjoy!

Nutritional Contents:

•Calories: 399

•Carbohydrate: 5.9 g

•Protein: 33 g

•Fat: 26.9 g

25

CHICKEN QUESADILLA

Prep Time: 10 minutes/ **Cook Time** 35 minutes/ **Serves:** 2

Ingredients :

•2 cups grilled chicken, sliced

•20 slices bacon, center-cut

•¼ cup ranch dressing

•½ cup cheddar cheese, shredded

Directions :

1.Preheat your Toaster Oven to 350 degrees F in toast mode

2.Line baking sheet using parchment paper

3.Weave bacon into two rectangles

4.Bake for 30 minutes

5.Lay grilled chicken over bacon square

6.Drizzle ranch dressing on top

7.Sprinkle cheddar cheese and top with another bacon square

8.Bake for 5 minutes more

9.Serve and enjoy!

Nutritional Contents:

•Calories: 37

•Carbohydrate: 2 g

- Protein: 1 g
- Fat: 3 g

26

DELICIOUS TURKEY CUTLETS

Prep Time: 10 minutes/ **Cook Time** 25 minutes/ **Serves:** 4

Ingredients :

•1 and ½ pounds turkey cutlets

•½ teaspoon onion powder

•1 egg

•½ teaspoon garlic powder

•¼ cup parmesan cheese, grated

•½ cup breadcrumbs

•½ teaspoon salt

•¼ teaspoon pepper

Directions :

1.Preheat your Oven t0 350 degrees F

2.Season turkey cutlets with salt and pepper

3.Add egg into a small bowl

4.Whisk it well

5.Take a shallow dish and add cheese, garlic powder, onion powder, and breadcrumbs

6.Dip the cutlet in the mixture

7.Coat them with breadcrumbs

8.Then bake for 25 minutes

9.Serve and enjoy!

Nutritional Contents:

•Calories: 398

•Carbohydrate: 10.4 g

•Protein: 56.1 g

•Fat: 12.6 g

27

TURKEY SPINACH PATTIES

Prep Time: 10 minutes/ **Cook Time** 30 minutes/ **Serves:** 4

Ingredients :

•1 pound turkey, grounded

•1/4 cup basil, chopped

•1 cup spinach, sauteed

•1 tablespoon olive oil

•2 tablespoons Worcestershire sauce

•1/4 cup breadcrumbs

•4 ounces mozzarella cheese, cubed

•1/4 cup parsley, chopped

•2 tablespoons vinegar

•1 teaspoon lemon zest

•1/2 onion, diced

•1 teaspoon garlic, minced

•Salt and pepper

Directions :

1.Preheat your Oven t0 350 degrees F

2.Take a large bowl and add all ingredients into it

3.Mix them until combine well

4.Make four patties from the mixture

5.Make sure the patties are in the same shape
6.Place them into baking pan
7.Then bake for 30-35 minutes
8.Serve and enjoy!

Nutritional Contents:

•Calories: 407
•Carbohydrate: 9.6 g
•Protein: 40.5 g
•Fat: 24.9 g

28

HEALTHY CHICKEN FRITTERS

Prep Time: 10 minutes/ **Cook Time** 25 minutes/ **Serves:** 4

Ingredients :

- •1 pound chicken, grounded
- •2 cups broccoli, cooked and chopped
- •1 and ½ cups mozzarella cheese, shredded
- •1 garlic clove, minced
- •¾ cup shallots, chopped
- •1 egg
- •¾ cup breadcrumbs
- •Salt and pepper

Directions :

1.Preheat your Oven t0 390 degrees F
2.Take a large bowl and add all ingredients into it
3.Mix them until combine well
4.Make small patties from the mixture
5.Place them onto the parchment-lined baking sheet
6.Then bake for 15 minutes
7.Flip them and bake for 10 minutes more
8.Serve and enjoy!

Nutritional Contents:

•Calories: 379

•Carbohydrate: 23.9 g

•Protein: 42 g

•Fat: 12.6 g

29

EASY BROWN SUGAR CHICKEN

Prep Time: 10 minutes/ **Cook Time** 30 minutes/ **Serves:** 4

Ingredients :

•4 chicken breasts, boneless and skinless

•1 tablespoon garlic, minced and sauteed

•¼ cup brown sugar

•Salt and pepper

Directions :

1.Preheat your Oven t0 450 degrees F

2.Take a casserole dish and spray cooking spray

3.Keep it aside

4.Season chicken breast with salt and pepper

5.Sprinkle over chicken

6.Place casserole dish onto the oven rack

7.Then bake for 25-30 minutes

8.Serve and enjoy!

Nutritional Contents:

•Calories: 345

•Carbohydrate: 9.6 g

•Protein: 42.5 g

•Fat: 14.3 g

SNACKS AND APPETIZERS

30

CINNAMON APPLE SLICES

Prep Time: 10 minutes/ **Cook Time** 30 minutes/ **Serves:** 4

Ingredients :

•3 apples, cut into ½ inch thick wedges

•2 tablespoons brown sugar

•1/3 cup butter, melted

•½ teaspoon cinnamon, grounded

Directions :

1.Preheat your Oven t0 350 degrees F

2.Add apple slices into the large mixing bowl

3.Take a small bowl and add melted butter, cinnamon, brown sugar, and sugar into it

4.Mix them well

5.Pour sugar mixture over apple slices

6.Mix them until it coated well

7.Place baking dish onto the oven rack

8.Then bake for 30 minutes

9.Stir apple slices after every 10 minutes

10.Serve and enjoy!

Nutritional Contents:

•Calories: 240
•Carbohydrate: 27.8 g
•Protein: 0.6 g
•Fat: 15.7 g

31

FLAX SEED CHIPS

Prep Time: 10 minutes/ **Cook Time** 15 minutes/ **Serves:** 4

Ingredients :

- ½ cup flax seeds
- 1 cup almond flour
- 1 teaspoon salt
- 1 and ½ teaspoons seasoned salt
- 1 pinch extra seasoned salt
- ½ cup of water

Directions :

1. Preheat your Toaster Oven to 330 degrees F
2. Take a container and add flax seeds, almond flour, sea salt, and 1 and ½ teaspoons seasoned salt into it
3. Stir in water up to the dough until mixed completely
4. Make the dough in narrow size, slices the size of a bite
5. Place them on a baking sheet
6. Sprinkle the rounds with seasoned salt
7. Bake for 15 minutes
8. Let it cool and store
9. Serve and enjoy!

Nutritional Contents:

•Calories: 126

•Carbohydrate: 15 g

•Protein: 2 g

•Fat: 6 g

32

TASTY ROASTED BROCCOLI

Prep Time: 5 minutes/ **Cook Time** 20 minutes/ **Serves:** 4

Ingredients :

•4 cups broccoli florets

•Sunflower seeds

•1 tablespoon olive oil

•Pepper, to taste

Directions :

1.Preheat your Oven to 400 degrees F in the Baking mode

2.Add broccoli in a zip bag alongside oil

3.Shake until coated

4.Add seasoning and shake again

5.Spread the broccoli out on the baking sheet

6.Bake for 20 minutes

7.Let it cool

8.Serve and enjoy!

Nutritional Contents:

•Calories: 62

•Carbohydrate: 4 g

•Protein: 4 g

•Fat: 4 g

33

HOME-MADE TRAIL MIX FOR THE TRIP

Prep Time: 10 minutes/ **Cook Time** 55 minutes/ **Serves:** 4

Ingredients :

•¼ cup almonds

•¼ cup walnuts

•2 tablespoons melted coconut oil

•¼ cup raw cashews

•1 teaspoon cinnamon

•Sunflower seeds as needed

Directions :

1.Preheat your Toaster Oven to 275 degrees F in toast mode

2.Line baking sheet with parchment paper

3.Melt coconut oil

4.Keep it on the side

5.Take a large mixing bowl and add nuts, cinnamon, and melted coconut oil

6.Stir it well

7.Sprinkle sunflower seeds

8.Place in Toaster Oven

9.Bake for 6 minutes

10.Serve and enjoy!

Nutritional Contents:

•Calories: 363

•Carbohydrate: 41 g

•Protein: 7 g

•Fat: 22 g

34

SPICY TARO CRUNCH

Prep Time: 10 minutes/ **Cook Time** 20 minutes/ **Serves:** 2

Ingredients :

- 2 cups taro, sliced thinly
- 1 teaspoon cayenne pepper powder
- 1 tablespoon olive oil
- A pinch salt

Directions :

1. Preheat your toaster oven to 350 degrees F in a toast mode
2. Add all the ingredients into a bowl
3. Toss to coat the taro with the spices and seasoning
4. Place the taro slices on a baking rack
5. Toast for 20 minutes
6. Serve and enjoy!

Nutritional Contents:

- Calories: 176
- Carbohydrate: 28 g
- Protein: 2 g
- Fat: 1 g

VEGAN AND VEGETARIAN

35

PERFECT POTATO CASSEROLE

Prep Time: 10 minutes/ **Cook Time** 35 minutes/ **Serves:** 10

Ingredients :

•20 ounces hash browns, diced

•1 pound sausage, cooked

•½ cup almond milk

•7 eggs

•8 ounces cheddar cheese, grated

•1 onion, chopped and sauteed

•Salt and pepper

Directions :

1.Preheat your Oven t0 350 degrees F

2.A spray casserole dish with cooking spray

3.Keep it aside

4.Add milk, whisked egg, salt, and pepper into a bowl

5.Then add the rest of the ingredients

6.Mix them well and set aside

7.Pour egg mixture into the prepared casserole dish

8.Place it into your over the rack

9.Bake for 35 minutes

10.Serve and enjoy!

Nutritional Contents:

•Calories: 393

•Carbohydrate: 18.5 g

•Protein: 17 g

•Fat: 27.8 g

36

ZUCCHINI TOMATO BAKE

Prep Time: 10 minutes/ **Cook Time** 30 minutes/ **Serves:** 6

Ingredients :

•2 medium zucchini, sliced

•½ cup parmesan cheese, shredded

•5 medium tomatoes, sliced

•½ teaspoon garlic powder

•2 medium yellow squash, sliced

•½ teaspoon Italian seasoning

•½ teaspoon onion powder

•½ teaspoon pepper

Directions :

1.Preheat your Oven t0 375 degrees F

2.Take your baking dish and grease it

3.Add zucchini, tomatoes, and squash in an alternating pattern

4.Top with cheese and spices

5.Then bake for 25-30 minutes

6.Serve and enjoy!

Nutritional Contents:

- Calories: 60
- Carbohydrate: 7 g
- Protein: 4.4 g
- Fat: 2.3 g

37

ZUCCHINI POTATO GRATIN

Prep Time: 10 minutes/ **Cook Time** 50 minutes/ **Serves:** 6

Ingredients :

- •1 and 1/2 zucchini, cut into 1/4 inch slices
- •1 cup Gruyere cheese, grated
- •5 small potatoes, cut into 1/8 inch slices
- •1 teaspoon herb de Provence
- •1 cup half and half
- •1 teaspoon garlic, minced
- •1 and 3/4 teaspoons salt
- •1/4 teaspoon pepper

Directions :

1.Preheat your Oven t0 400 degrees F
2.Take an 8* 6-inch baking dish and grease it
3.Arrange vegetables in a circular pattern into the dish
4.Add herb de Provence, half and half, garlic, salt and pepper
5.Mix them well and pour over the vegetables
6.Sprinkle grated cheese on top
7.Then bake for 50 minutes
8.Serve and enjoy!

Nutritional Contents:

•Calories: 256

•Carbohydrate: 31 g

•Protein: 6 g

•Fat: 6 g

38

GARLIC CHEESE DIP

Prep Time: 10 minutes/ **Cook Time** 20 minutes/ **Serves:** 6

Ingredients :

•1 teaspoon garlic, minced

•¼ cup parmesan cheese, shredded

•½ cup mozzarella cheese, shredded

•2 cups ricotta cheese

•1 lemon zest

•3 tablespoons olive oil

•Salt and pepper

Directions :

1.Preheat your Oven t0 375 degrees F

2.Add all the ingredients into the bowl

3.Mix to combine well

4.Pour the mixture into the greased casserole dish

5.Place the casserole dish onto the oven rack

6.Then bake for 20 minutes

7.Serve and enjoy!

Nutritional Contents:

•Calories: 181

- Carbohydrate: 4.5 g
- Protein: 10.1 g
- Fat: 14 g

39

BAKED POTATO WEDGES

Prep Time: 10 minutes/ **Cook Time** 15 minutes/ **Serves:** 4

Ingredients :

•2 potatoes, cut into wedges

•½ teaspoon garlic powder

•½ teaspoon paprika

•1/8 teaspoon chili powder

•2 tablespoons olive oil

•Salt

Directions :

1.Preheat your Oven t0 350 degrees F

2.Soak potato wedges in the water for 1 hour

3.Drain the water and pat dry by using a towel

4.Take a bowl and add garlic powder, paprika, potato wedges with oil, chili powder, and salt into it

5.Spread potato wedges on the parchment-lined baking pan

6.Bake for 15-20 minutes

7.Serve and enjoy!

Nutritional Contents:

•Calories: 136

•Carbohydrate: 17.2 g
•Protein: 1.9 g
•Fat: 7.2 g

40

STUFFED BELL PEPPER

Prep Time: 10 minutes/ **Cook Time** 10 minutes/ **Serves:** 2

Ingredients :

•4 bell peppers, halved and hollowed

•½ cup baby spinach

•12 black olives, halved

•2 garlic cloves, minced

•½ cup quinoa, cooked

•1/3 cup tomatoes, sun-dried

•Salt and pepper for taste

Directions :

1.Preheat your Toaster Oven to 400 degrees F in toast mode

2.Take a bowl and all the ingredients except bell pepper

3.Mix them well

4.Bake for 10 minutes

5.Once cooked, stuff pepper with quinoa mixture

6.Serve and enjoy!

Nutritional Contents:

•Calories: 126

•Carbohydrate: 19 g

- Protein: 3 g
- Fat: 5 g

41

BAKED CURRIED CAULIFLOWER FLORETS

Prep Time: 10 minutes/ **Cook Time** 15 minutes/ **Serves:** 4

Ingredients :

- 2 pounds cauliflower, cut into florets
- 2 teaspoons fresh lemon juice
- 1 teaspoon kosher salt
- 1 and ½ teaspoons curry powder
- 1 tablespoon olive oil

Directions :

1. Preheat your Oven t0 425 degrees F
2. Toss cauliflower florets with oil, salt, and curry powder
3. Spread cauliflower florets onto the baking sheet
4. Bake for 15 minutes
5. Drizzle lemon juice on top
6. Serve and enjoy!

Nutritional Contents:

- Calories: 90
- Carbohydrate: 12 g
- Protein: 4 g
- Fat: 4 g

42

BALSAMIC MUSHROOMS

Prep Time: 10 minutes/ **Cook Time** 20 minutes/ **Serves:** 6

Ingredients :

•1 pound button mushrooms, scrubbed

•½ teaspoon oregano, diced

•1 tablespoon garlic, crushed

•2 tablespoons olive oil

•4 tablespoons balsamic vinegar

•½ teaspoon basil, dried

•¼ teaspoon black pepper

•1 teaspoon of sea salt

Directions :

1.Preheat your Oven t0 425 degrees F

2.Take a mixing bowl and add all the ingredients

3.Mix them well

4.Spread mushrooms onto the baking sheet

5.Bake for 20 minutes

6.Serve and enjoy!

Nutritional Contents:

•Calories: 60

- •Carbohydrate: 3 g
- •Protein: 2.5 g
- •Fat: 5 g

43

ZUCCHINI CHIPS

Prep Time: 10 minutes/ **Cook Time** 5 hours/ **Serves:** 4

Ingredients :

•2 zucchinis, sliced thinly

•1/4 teaspoon chili powder

•Salt

•1/4 teaspoon paprika, smoked

Directions :

1.Take a bowl and add zucchini slices, chili powder, smoked paprika, and salt to it

2.Toss them well

3.Place a rack onto a baking tray

4.Then arrange zucchini slices onto the rack

5.Insert into the Oven

6.Set the Dehydrate mode

7.Set the timer for 5 hours

8.Serve and enjoy!

Nutritional Contents:

•Calories: 17

•Carbohydrate: 3.4 g

- Protein: 1.2 g
- Fat: 0.2 g

44

BANANA SLICES

Prep Time: 10 minutes/ **Cook Time** 5 hours/ **Serves:** 4

Ingredients :

•4 bananas, peel and cut into 1/8 inch slices

Directions :

1.Place a rack onto a baking tray

2.Then arrange banana slices onto the rack

3.Insert into the Oven

4.Set the Dehydrate mode

5.Set the timer for 5 hours

6.Serve and enjoy!

Nutritional Contents:

•Calories: 105

•Carbohydrate: 27 g

•Protein: 1.3 g

•Fat: 0.4 g

45

LOVELY ROASTED BAMBOO SPROUTS

Prep Time: 10 minutes/ **Cook Time** 15 minutes/ **Serves:** 3

Ingredients :

•1 pound bamboo sprouts

•1 cup cashew cheese

•¼ teaspoon paprika

•2 tablespoons almond butter

•Salt and pepper to taste

Directions :

1.Preheat your Toaster Oven to 350 degrees F in toast mode

2.Take a baking dish

3.Grease the dish with oil

4.Take a bowl and add butter, salt, pepper, paprika to it

5.Mix them well

6.Add bamboo to the butter marinade, mix well

7.Marinate for 1 hour

8.Transfer to a baking dish

9.Bake for 15 minutes

10.Serve and enjoy!

Nutritional Contents:

- Calories: 192
- Carbohydrate: 2 g
- Protein: 12 g
- Fat: 15 g

BEANS AND EGGS

46

FLUFFY BREAKFAST EGG MUFFINS

Prep Time: 10 minutes/ **Cook Time** 25 minutes/ **Serves:** 12

Ingredients :

•12 eggs

•½ cup cheddar cheese, shredded

•½ cup almond milk

•¼ teaspoon garlic powder

•½ cup ham, diced

•Salt and pepper

Directions :

1.Preheat your Oven t0 375 degrees F

2.Spray 12-cups muffin tin with cooking spray

3.Keep it aside

4.Add whisked eggs, garlic powder, milk, salt, and pepper into a bowl

5.Add cheese and ham

6.Stir it well

7.Pour egg mixture into the prepared muffin tin

8.Place it into your over the rack

9.Bake for 25 minutes

10.Serve and enjoy!

Nutritional Contents:

•Calories: 114

•Carbohydrate: 1.2 g

•Protein: 7.9 g

•Fat: 8.8 g

47

TURMERIC SCRAMBLED EGGS

Prep Time: 10 minutes/ **Cook Time** 15 minutes/ **Serves:** 4

Ingredients:

•8-10 eggs, large and pasture-raised

•1 teaspoon cilantro, chopped

•½ teaspoon turmeric powder

•½ cup almond or coconut milk, unsweetened

•¼ teaspoon black pepper

•A pinch salt

Directions:

1.Preheat your toaster oven to 350 degrees F, in bake mode

2.Take a casserole or heat-proof baking dish and grease

3.Take a bowl and whisk eggs, black pepper, turmeric powder, milk, and salt

4.Pour the mixture into the baking dish

5.Transfer baking dish to the Oven and bake for 15 minutes until the eggs have set

6.Remove from Oven

7.Garnish with chopped cilantro if desired

8.Enjoy!

Nutritional Contents:
•Calories: 203
•Fat: 16g
•Carbohydrates: 5g
•Protein: 10g

48

BAKED ARTICHOKE AND EGGS

Prep Time: 10 minutes/ **Cook Time** 20 minutes/ **Serves:** 4

Ingredients:

•4 whole eggs

•4 slices low-fat cheddar, shredded

•1 yellow onion, chopped

•1 tablespoon avocado oil

•1 tablespoon cilantro, chopped

•1 cup canned no salt added artichokes, drained and chopped

Directions:

1.Grease 4 ramekins with oil, divide onion in each

2.Crack an egg into each ramekin

3.Add artichokes and top with cilantro, cheddar cheese

4.Transfer ramekins to Toaster Oven, bake for 20 minutes at 380 degrees F in Bake Mode

5.Serve and enjoy!

Nutritional Contents:

•Calories: 446

•Fat: 29g

•Carbohydrates: 37g

•Protein: 13g

49

SALAMI AND PROSCIUTTO EGG BAKE

Prep Time: 10 minutes/ **Cook Time** 15 minutes/ **Serves:** 4

Ingredients:

•½ teaspoon onion powder

•4 eggs, beaten

•1 cup mozzarella cheese, grated

•3 ounces salami, chopped

•4 slices prosciutto, chopped

•1 beef sausage, chopped

Directions:

1.Preheat Toaster Oven on Bake function to 350 F.

2.Whisk the eggs with the onion powder—Brown the sausage in a skillet over medium heat for 2 minutes.

3.Remove the egg mixture and add in mozzarella cheese, salami, and prosciutto and stir it.

4.Pour the egg mixture into a greased baking pan and cook for 10-15 minutes until golden brown on top. Serve.

Nutritional Contents:

•Calories: 154

•Fat: 10g

•Carbohydrates: 1g
•Protein: 17g

50

CHILI BEAN BURRITO

Prep Time: 10 minutes/ **Cook Time** 5 minutes/ **Serves:** 4

Ingredients:

•1 teaspoon Italian seasoning

•1 can – 8 ounces beans

•1 cup cheddar cheese, grated

•6 tortillas

Directions:

1.Preheat Toaster Oven on Bake function to 350 F.

2.Season the beans with the seasoning and divide them between the tortillas.

3.Top with cheddar cheese.

4.Roll the burritos and arrange them on a lined baking dish—Cook for 5 minutes. Serve.

Nutritional Contents:

•Calories: 590

•Fat: 25g

•Carbohydrates: 71g

•Protein: 24g

51

GARBANZO BEAN MEAL

Prep Time: 10 minutes/ **Cook Time** 25 minutes/ **Serves:** 4

Ingredients:

- 1 can garbanzo beans, chickpeas
- 1 tablespoon olive oil
- 1 teaspoon sunflower seeds
- 1 teaspoon garlic powder
- ½ teaspoon paprika

Directions:

1. Preheat your Toaster Oven to 375 degrees F in Bake Mode
2. Line a baking sheet with a silicone baking mat
3. Drain and rinse garbanzo beans, pat garbanzo beans dry, and pout into a large bowl
4. Toss with olive oil, sunflower seeds, garlic powder, paprika and mix well
5. Spread over a baking sheet
6. Bake for 20 minutes at 375 degrees F
7. Turn chickpeas, so they are roasted well
8. Place back in Toaster Oven and bake for 25 minutes at 375 degrees F
9. Let them cool and enjoy!

Nutritional Contents:

•Calories: 178

•Fat: 25g

•Carbohydrates: 366g

•Protein: 25g

52

ZUCCHINI AND BLACK BEAN ENCHILADA

Prep Time: 10 minutes/ **Cook Time** 20 minutes/ **Serves:** 4

Ingredients:

- •3 large zucchini, diced
- •1 cup black beans, cooked
- •1 cup tomatoes, diced
- •1 and 1/4 teaspoon garlic salt
- •3 teaspoons extra virgin olive oil
- •1/4 cup goat cheese, diced
- •1/2 small red onion, chopped
- •A handful of coriander, chopped
- •Salt and pepper, to taste

Directions:

1.Preheat your toaster oven to 375 degrees F in Bake Mode

2.Take a baking tray and place zucchini and drizzle with olive oil

3.Season with garlic salt

4.Bake for 20 minutes

5.Let it cool

6.Take a bowl and combine all ingredients into the bowl

7.Serve with vegetable chips and enjoy!

Nutritional Contents:
•Calories: 225
•Fat: 9g
•Carbohydrates: 22g
•Protein: 14g

53

BAKED EGGS WITH PORTOBELLO MUSHROOMS

Prep Time: 10 minutes/ **Cook Time** 20 minutes/ **Serves:** 4

Ingredients :

•4 portobello mushroom caps

•1 medium tomato, chopped

•1 cup arugula

•4 large eggs, pasture-raised

•Salt and pepper, to taste

Directions :

1.Preheat your Oven t0 350 degrees F

2.Line a baking sheet with parchment paper

3.Scoop out the gills first and then discard the gills

4.Set it aside

5.Place the mushrooms on the baking sheet inverted

6.Fill with arugula and tomato

7.Add an egg to each mushroom cap

8.Bake for 20 minutes

9.Serve and enjoy!

Nutritional Contents:

•Calories: 83

- Carbohydrate: 5 g
- Protein: 5 g
- Fat: 5 g

54

TOMATO AND FETA OLIVE TART

Prep Time: 10 minutes/ **Cook Time** 15-20 minutes/ **Serves:** 4

Ingredients:

•4 whole eggs

•Salt and pepper to taste

•½ cup milk

•2 tablespoon olive oil

•¼ cup onion, chopped

•¼ cup Kalamata olives, chopped

•1 tablespoon fresh oregano, chopped

•1 tablespoon fresh basil, chopped

•1 cup feta cheese, crumbled

Directions:

1.Preheat Toaster oven on Bake function to 360 degrees F

2.Brush a pie pan with olive oil. Beat the eggs along with the milk, salt, and pepper.

3.Stir in all of the remaining ingredients. Pour the egg mixture into the pan—Cook for 20 minutes.

Nutritional Contents:

- Calories: 583
- Fat: 32g
- Carbohydrates: 49g
- Protein: 26g

DESSERTS AND SNACKS

55

PUMPKIN BREAD

Prep Time: 10 minutes/ **Cook Time** 35 minutes/ **Serves:** 8

Ingredients :

•½ cup pumpkin puree

•1 teaspoon pumpkin pie spice

•¼ cup of chocolate chips

•2 eggs

•¼ cup coconut flour

•¼ cup flax seed meal

•¼ cup Swerve

•1 teaspoon baking powder

Directions :

1.Preheat your Oven t0 350 degrees F

2.Grease loaf pan with

3.Set them aside

4.Add all the dry ingredients into the bowl

5.Mix them well and keep aside

6.Add eggs and whisked pumpkin puree into another bowl

7.Then add wet ingredients mixture into dry ingredients

8.Mix to combine well

9.Pour the batter into the prepared loaf pan

10.Place it into your over the rack
11.Bake for 35 minutes
12.Serve and enjoy!

Nutritional Contents:

•Calories: 69
•Carbohydrate: 5.9 g
•Protein: 2.6 g
•Fat: 3.8 g

56

HEALTHY BANANA BREAD

Prep Time: 10 minutes/ **Cook Time** 55 minutes/ **Serves:** 12

Ingredients :

•3 bananas, ripe

•1 teaspoon baking soda

•2 cups flour

•1/4 teaspoon cinnamon, grounded

•1 cup of sugar

•2 eggs

•1 teaspoon vanilla

•1 stick butter, melted

•1/2 teaspoon salt

Directions :

1.Preheat your Oven t0 350 degrees F

2.Take a mixing bowl and add melted butter and bananas into it

3.Mash them with a fork

4.Then add vanilla and eggs, stir well

5.Add baking soda, cinnamon, flour, sugar, and salt into another bowl

6.Add flour mixture to the banana mixture

7.Pour batter into the greased 9* 5-inch loaf pan
8.Place the pan onto the oven rack
9.Bake for 45-55 minutes
10.Serve and enjoy!

Nutritional Contents:

•Calories: 244
•Carbohydrate: 39.5 g
•Protein: 3.5 g
•Fat: 8.7 g

57

CINNAMON HONEY PEARS

Prep Time: 10 minutes/ **Cook Time** 30 minutes/ **Serves:** 4

Ingredients :

•4 pears, peel, cut in ½ and scoop out and core

•½ teaspoon vanilla

•½ teaspoon cinnamon, grounded

•2 tablespoons butter, melted

•3 tablespoons honey

Directions :

1.Preheat your Oven t0 400 degrees F

2.Take a 9* 13-inch baking dish and place pears

3.Take a small bowl and add honey, cinnamon, melted butter, and vanilla to it

4.Pour honey mixture over pears

5.Place baking dish onto the oven rack

6.Then bake for 30 minutes

7.Once done, allow it cool for 5-10 minutes

8.Serve and enjoy!

Nutritional Contents:

•Calories: 222

- Carbohydrate: 45.1 g
- Protein: 0.9 g
- Fat: 6.1 g

58

MOIST YOGURT CAKE

Prep Time: 10 minutes/ **Cook Time** 40 minutes/ **Serves:** 8

Ingredients :

•1 cup plain yogurt

•2 eggs

•2 teaspoons baking powder

•½ cup canola oil

•½ cup sugar 2 cups all-purpose flour

•1 lemon zest

•½ teaspoon vanilla

•3 tablespoons orange jam

•Pinch of salt

Directions :

1.Preheat your Oven t0 350 degrees F

2.Take a 9.5* 2.5-inch loaf pan and grease it

3.Keep it aside

4.Add eggs, vanilla, lemon zest, yogurt, sugar, and oil into a mixing bowl

5.Beat them until smooth

6.Add flour, baking powder, salt, and mix until just combined

7.Pour batter into the prepared loaf pan

8.Place loaf pan onto the oven rack

9.Add apple slices into the large mixing bowl

10.Then bake for 35-40 minutes

11.Once cooked, removed the pan and allow it to cool for 10 minutes

12.Add orange jam on top of the cake

13.Serve and enjoy!

Nutritional Contents:

•Calories: 321

•Carbohydrate: 39.2 g

•Protein: 6.4 g

•Fat: 15.4 g

59

SOFT AND MOIST LEMON BROWNIE

Prep Time: 10 minutes/ **Cook Time** 20 minutes/ **Serves:** 16

Ingredients :

•¾ cup all-purpose flour

•½ cup butter softened

•2 eggs

•½ teaspoon baking powder

•½ lemon zest

•1 tablespoon fresh lemon juice

•¾ cup of sugar

Directions :

1.Preheat your Oven t0 350 degrees F

2.Take an 8* 8-inch baking pan

3.Keep it aside

4.Take a large bowl and add butter, lemon zest, and sugar to it

5.Beat them until it gets fluffy

6.Add eggs, lemon juice, and flour

7.Mix well

8.Pour the batter into the prepared pan and spread evenly

9.Place the pan onto the oven rack

10.Then bake for 20 minutes

11. Once cooked, removed the pan and allow it to cool
12. Serve and enjoy!

Nutritional Contents:

- Calories: 116
- Carbohydrate: 14 g
- Protein: 1.4 g
- Fat: 6.4 g

60

EASY BLONDE BROWNIE

Prep Time: 10 minutes/ **Cook Time** 40 minutes/ **Serves:** 8

Ingredients :

•2 cups all-purpose flour

•2 teaspoons baking powder

•2 eggs

•½ cup of chocolate chips

•1 cup butter, melted

•1 and ½ teaspoon vanilla

•1 and ¼ cups brown sugar

•½ teaspoon salt

Directions :

1.Preheat your Oven t0 350 degrees F

2.Take a 9* 13-inch baking pan

3.Keep it aside

4.Take a mixing bowl and add melted butter, vanilla, eggs, and sugar into it

5.Mix them well

6.Add flour, baking powder, and salt

7.Mix until well combined

8.Add chocolate chips and stir well

9.Pour the batter into the prepared pan and spread evenly
10.Place the pan onto the oven rack
11.Then bake for 20 minutes
12.Once cooked, removed the pan and allow it to cool
13.Serve and enjoy!

Nutritional Contents:

•Calories: 479
•Carbohydrate: 53.1 g
•Protein: 5.7 g
•Fat: 27.5 g

61

HEALTHY TAHINI BUNS

Prep Time: 10 minutes/ **Cook Time** 15-20 minutes/ **Serves:** 3

Ingredients :

•1 whole egg

•5 tablespoons Tahini paste

•½ teaspoon baking soda

•1 teaspoon lemon juice

•1 pinch salt

Directions :

1.Preheat your Toaster Oven to 350 degrees F in toast mode

2.Line baking sheet with parchment paper

3.Add all the listed ingredients to a blender

4.Blend until you get a smooth batter

5.Scoop batter onto prepared sheet forming buns

6.Bake for 15-20 minutes

7.Once done, remove from Toaster Oven and let them cool

8.Serve and enjoy!

Nutritional Contents:

•Calories: 172

- Carbohydrate: 7 g
- Protein: 6 g
- Fat: 14 g

62

CREATIVE CINNAMON BREAD

Prep Time: 10 minutes/ **Cook Time** 25-30 minutes/ **Serves:** 10

Ingredients :

•3 eggs, pastured
•½ teaspoon baking soda
•1 teaspoon cinnamon
•½ teaspoon baking powder
•1 teaspoon vinegar
•1/3 cup pure sour cream
•1/8 teaspoon stevia
•3 tablespoons salted butter
•2 tablespoons water
•½ cup coconut flour

Directions :

1.Preheat your Toaster Oven to 350 degrees F in Bake Mode
2.Take a loaf pan and grease it with oil
3.Line the bottom with parchment paper
4.Mix dry ingredients in a bowl
5.Whisk them well
6.Add remaining ingredients to the dry mix and mix well

7.Taste for sweetness
8.Adjust seasoning
9.Keep it aside for 3 minutes
10.Spread batter onto the loaf pan
11.Bake for 25-30 minutes
12.Allow it to cool before serving
13.Serve and enjoy!

Nutritional Contents:

•Calories: 468
•Carbohydrate: 17 g
•Protein: 11 g
•Fat: 45 g

AFTERWORD

I can't express how honored I am to think that you found my book interesting and informative enough to read it all through to the end.

Thank you again for purchasing this book, and I hope that you had as much fun reading it as I had writing it.

I bid you farewell and encourage you to move forward in your journey with the Luby French Door Toaster Oven and pray that you find success in your quest!

Lightning Source UK Ltd.
Milton Keynes UK
UKHW021549030321
379704UK00005B/25

9 781801 726061